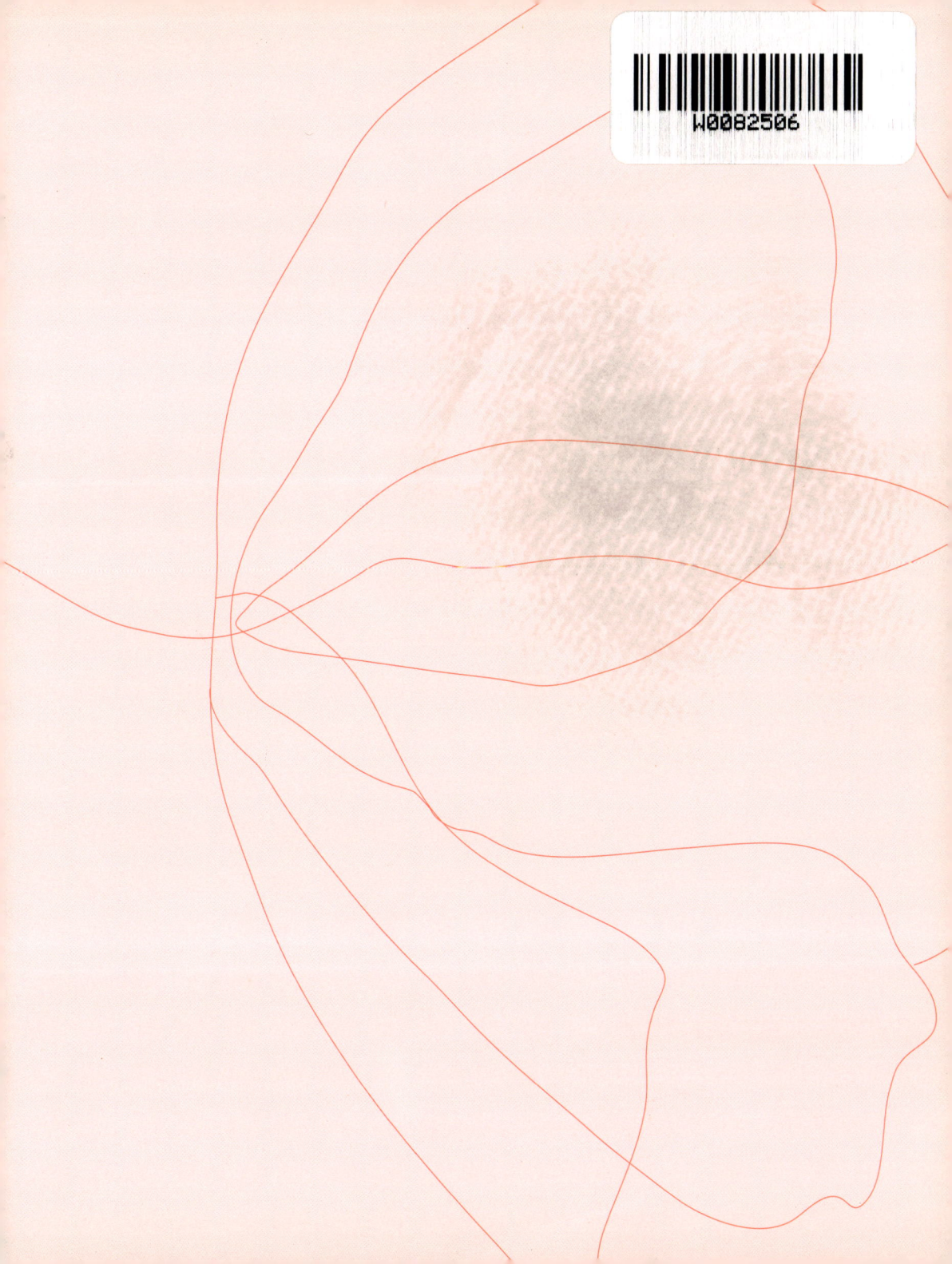

THIS BOOK BELONGS TO

....

INTRODUCTION

Welcome to your new pregnancy journal, Mama!

This is exciting! So, where to begin? Let's begin with YOU. Perhaps this journal finds you right at the start of your pregnancy as you begin your progression through the three trimesters and all the changes that they will bring. If that's the case, then it's good to know that you have all this space to write about your very first inklings and to note down every detail all the way through this special phase of life, recording precious things that might otherwise be forgotten in the months ahead when you have a little baby to care for.

But as many pregnancies are only discovered a month or two into the process, maybe it has arrived into your hands when your pregnancy is already well underway? If so, there may be past moments that you wish you could have captured at the time, so please remember you can always write these down in retrospect as you go through the book. Obviously these pages are yours and you can use them as and however you like; you don't need to follow my prompts or even use the time-frame offered here. Just claim the journal for yourself and for your own needs, wishes and expressions.

Having said that, you might like to consider how you want to use this book to really enjoy and get the most out of it. It could be helpful to imagine yourself in ten years' time, and think to yourself... 'What would I want to remember about my life at this time?'

Maybe you could think of your pregnancy journal a bit like starting a new relationship, with a warm and patient friend who loves to listen, without judging, who can hear your bright moods as well as your stormy ones, your joys and hopes as well as your fears and doubts. A friend who can receive all of YOU with kindness and spaciousness.

This little book you are holding could be your sanctuary during your pregnancy; your safe space to explore and unravel the multifaceted aspects of a mother's, or mother-to-be's, life – both your inner and your outer life, as you experience gestation, childbirth and beyond. My feeling is that pregnancy is like an incubation time for women, during which so much change happens. It is really special to consciously reflect on how you might be changing, or on how you might wish to change. Because when we, as mothers, give birth to our new children we will also be giving birth to ourselves anew in some way. It is unavoidable. The act of birthing and mothering a new child, or more than one child, cannot help but transform us even if we are mothers already. And this can be a deeply positive experience when we embrace it wholeheartedly with both the softness and edges it brings.

My wish is for this journal to support you as you transition from woman to mother or from mother into motherhood again. It is a remarkable journey, only made 'ordinary' by the fact that it happens to women every day. But the path of motherhood is both physiologically and emotionally complex, sophisticated and truly incredible. And as it changes us collectively as women, so the children we give birth to, will in some way change the planet forever too, generation by generation. It's BIG stuff we are doing!

So please do not underestimate yourself and your path as a mother. Your experience is as important as your wellbeing, and I hope that you find some nourishment, joy and strength as you write in the pages before you. In this busy world that we inhabit, just taking some time to devote to yourself, to say what YOU have to say, and explore what YOU are feeling or thinking, can bring small moments of release or insights that might just relieve your stress and make your life sweeter in some way. Pregnancy should include these moments of sweetness, of calm, of recognition and understanding. And if that isn't happening so far then it's good to find ways of making it happen.

Whether this is your first baby or you are already an old hand at motherhood, each pregnancy like each child has its own unique character and can never be repeated. So by making use of this time to keep a journal and reflect on your life, you will have a written reminder of this particular pregnancy and you will be creating something that you can always treasure.

THE FIRST TRIMESTER

So here we go...

We'll start at the beginning, where all pregnancies start, with the huge hormonal changes and shifts going on inside us, that can give rise to all kinds of feelings, both physical and emotional. More rapid physical change and growth happens for your child during their life in your womb than at any other time in their whole lives. The first eight weeks after conception are called the embryonic stage, during which time they develop from a single cell into a tiny foetus with skeleton, limbs, nervous system and all major organs. Isn't that amazing? It's certainly an inspirational thing to remember as you are hunched over the sink with morning sickness!

It may be that the tiny form developing inside you is much smaller than a pea, but the reality is that its presence in your womb is having a huge impact. And the high-dose mélange of hormones orchestrating the rapid development of this little sweet pea may be ruffling your feathers big time. You might be going through everything from nausea and loss of appetite to an unlimited growth in appetite; from feelings of sadness to feelings of expansiveness and joy. Each of us will have our own personal response to those first few weeks of change in our physical chemistry, and there is no way of telling how it's going to be before it happens. But when it does happen, we are certainly going to have something to say about it. And that is where these pages come into their own – as your own private space in which to respond to your inner thoughts.

Connecting with your womb and your growing little one...

As mothers and mothers-to-be, the focus is on 'managing' pregnancy's first phase as we adjust to the ongoing changes. This can be more intense for some women and less so for others. But either way it might be helpful to practise putting your hands on your womb when you find time, and just to breathe into your belly and try to connect with this tiny new cellular presence inside you.

Do you observe anything? If so, what? And if not, you can use this space to explore how you feel about this little embryo being inside you...

Early Days

There is so much going on in your womb in the first month of pregnancy. After the process of fertilization is completed, cellular construction gets under way! The fertilized egg begins as one cell and quickly divides, cell by cell, into a cluster of individual cells called a morula, (or 'mulberry', a microscopically small one!) within your original egg.

This soon transforms into a larger blastocyst as it floats around in your uterine fluid. When it is around 150 cells strong, it begins to organize itself into the interior cells, which will become your baby, and the outside cells, which will become the placenta and amniotic sac. Now it is ready to snuggle into the wall of your uterus and be nourished. It produces little 'villi' roots, which embed themselves in the wall and draw molecules of oxygen, protein, sugars and other essential nutrients from it to feed the ever-evolving cluster of cells. By about Week Four, it gradually becomes a tiny embryo.

As most pregnancies aren't discovered until after this month, the few pages here are for your reflections on this initial phase, and will most probably be written in retrospect.

So this space is for you to record those first dawning notions...

What made you think you could be pregnant? Do you remember where you were?

....

....

....

....

....

....

....

....

What were your first thoughts or feelings? What did you do?

....

....

....

....

....

....

....

....

....

....

....

When did you know for sure and who did you tell first?

....

....

....

....

What were your initial pregnancy 'symptoms'?

....

....

....

....

....

....

....

....

....

Did you notice physical changes or intense moods?

....

....

....

....

....

....

....

....

....

Did you experience any cravings or aversions to food and drink?

....

....

....

....

....

....

....

....

How long did it take for your pregnancy to sink in for you?

Was it a surprise or a planned pregnancy?

Did you feel prepared or unprepared?

Adjustment and attunement

When we become pregnant we embark on a journey of adjustment and attunement that will last in different ways throughout all of our child's phases of growth towards adulthood. In pregnancy we are at some level adjusting our lives to meet our new circumstantial needs. These may be subtle or distinct changes in our diet, our choice of clothing, and perhaps our actions. Many of us feel extremely tired in the first trimester and we might start to become aware of what we feel physically comfortable or uncomfortable with doing at a given time.

We may decide to give up drinking or smoking to protect our growing baby. We may make some clear alterations to our practical lives, and alongside these hands-on responses to being pregnant, we will also in some way be attuning to our pregnancy – and later on, to our baby, and beyond this, to our child. What I mean by attunement is following our instinctual and empathic sense of things.

Pregnancy and into early motherhood is a hormone-fuelled time when women can perhaps feel more sensitivity, empathy and clear gut-instinct than during other phases of life. Developing this capacity and learning how to deeply trust oneself is a great thing.

So here are some pages for you to think about the adjustments you are making during this formative stage and to find words for some of the feelings, urges and instinctual responses you have as a newly pregnant woman.

What adjustments have you made already?

....
....
....
....
....
....
....
....

What adjustments do you think you still need to make?

....
....
....
....
....
....
....
....
....

Explain your feelings, urges and instinctual responses to being pregnant?

....
....
....
....
....
....
....

Dreams

Dreams during pregnancy can be both vivid and fascinating, and they'll be lovely to look back on in the years to come. So as you journal through this book, please don't forget to include your dreams in this space. Especially if you have been taking a bit more time out to rest and have the chance to dream more, do write about them and record what you think they might represent for you and the feelings that they evoke for you.

Can you remember any recent dreams?

Dreams during
pregnancy can
be both vivid
and fascinating

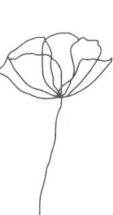

What's happening in your womb-world?

In the second month of pregnancy your little embryo grows from around 2 millimetres to 13 millimetres long. During Weeks 5 and 6 it begins to develop a nervous system. Its heart starts to beat and blood vessels in the evolving umbilical cord connect the heart to the placenta. Throughout Weeks 6 to 8 there is a rapid expansion in cellular growth during which your embryo transitions from a tadpole-like form into a tiny human being with the early stages of eyes, ears, mouth and limbs. It lies within a sac that already contains amniotic fluid and receives all of its nourishment from your placenta.

By Week 8 you may be feeling tired if you weren't before. You may find yourself catching your breath more often, because your circulation now has more to do, and you may be peeing more due to your increased kidney flow. Additional hormones can also cause constipation at this time, too, so eating fibrous foods will support your digestive system now. Putting grated beetroot into a salad or soaking flax or chia seeds and adding these to your muesli are fantastically easy ways to stay regular.

Folic acid and a good prenatal vitamin are really important supplements for your nutrition right now, especially if you're feeling too nauseous to eat a varied diet. Just eat what you can and try not to give yourself a hard time about it. But the more fresh and nutritious your ingredients are, the happier your body will be overall. If you can only manage toast for now, don't worry, you can always make up for lost time later when your nausea subsides by eating the healthiest diet on the planet. It is good to remember that for many women the first trimester is the most challenging phase of pregnancy and things very often get easier from here on.

So how do you feel in your pregnancy right now?

Start by describing how your body feels and any physical sensations you have experienced.

What changes have you noticed in your body so far?

Have there been any changes to your mood or emotions?

Explore how you feel about your changing body and your pregnancy 'symptoms'?

What do you need?

What do you feel that you need to support your body, heart and mind? Be generous with yourself. If you need more quiet time each day just to sit and rest, or a daytime nap, or particular foods, or lovely visits with your favourite people, explore how this could look for you. Your body is hard at work making a baby, so think about ways of giving to yourself and supporting your own progress all the way.

What do you feel you need to support yourself through this pregnancy?

Third month

As your pregnancy becomes more established in month three,
the small being inside you evolves from embryo to foetus, becoming
more 'baby-like' by the moment. Your body is likely to be looking
or feeling a little more pregnant at this stage and you might begin
to sense everything starting to 'settle in'. Nausea tends to wear off
between Weeks 10 to 14, which comes as a huge relief to those who
experience 'morning sickness'. With the understanding that everything
is looking positive for your pregnancy, it can be really useful to take
stock of your experience thus far. Let's start with the negatives first so
that we can then move on to the positives.

CHALLENGES

This space is for all your grumbles or anything that has riled you over
the last 3 months. It is a space for you to rant if you want to, to vent
your spleen or simply to explore anything that you feel is missing or
tricky about your life right now.

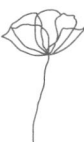

Thanks for giving that up! Sometimes having a moan is really important, it can help us to crystallize issues that are lying low and need to be addressed, or simply help us to let off steam. If you need more than one page, find somewhere else to continue writing. Don't stop just because the paper runs out if you have more to say!

GRATITUDE

Here we come to expressing what you feel gratitude for. Just list the wonderful and good things in your life at the moment. This is both a great practice for times when you may be feeling low, or equally for those times when you feel that your cup is brimming over!

You may want to close your eyes and take a few breaths here before naming all the people and things you feel grateful for.

CELEBRATE!

And finally, let's celebrate! This is an important part of motherhood. We are going to find ourselves recognizing and praising our babies and children when they achieve something like smiling, rolling over or mastering how to hold a spoon to feed themselves, and when they begin to speak or walk. If we can begin to notice our own achievements in pregnancy, or to step back and acknowledge the significant events in our lives, we will be creating a positive mindset that can sustain us through the adversities, as well as magnifying the enjoyable aspects of all that lies ahead.

The reality is that when we celebrate our lives, we become more resilient. So this is a space for you to celebrate in words anything you like from your First Trimester.

Beginning to notice
your own achievements
in pregnancy creates a
positive mindset that
can sustain you through
adversities

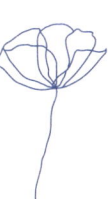

THE SECOND TRIMESTER

When people speak of a pregnant woman 'blooming' or 'glowing', it often begins in this phase of pregnancy – hopefully you'll be feeling a bit like a goddess. During the second trimester we tend to feel energized in a grounded way and physically strong – some women use the term 'invincible' – with those pregnancy hormones potent in our blood. Obviously we will still get tired out, and our energy reserves need to be respected and used carefully, but if we are eating and resting well and avoiding stress, this can be the loveliest time.

As your belly becomes fuller, your pregnancy may start to feel like more of a reality; that there actually is a little being in there making its short-term, formative home in your womb. In fact, this being is growing rapidly, forming fingernails, ears, nose and eyes. Its skeleton is starting to become distinct and harder than the rest of its surrounding body and its reproductive organs are taking shape. So, if you are having your scan at around 20 weeks, it will be possible to tell whether you're carrying a baby girl or boy (just remember to tell the midwives if you don't want to know).

Health & Community

If you haven't done any antenatal yoga classes yet, this could be the best time to dive in and support your physical body's tone and naturally increasing suppleness, while getting all the benefits of breathing exercises that calm the mind in preparation for the time leading up to, during and after giving birth. It is also an excellent way to connect with other mums and mums-to-be as you are likely to see each other regularly and can share together in your stages and phases of pregnancy.

Women are wonderful community builders, we just do it naturally, and having a community of mothers around you is an important part of this journey. It's very valuable to have friends who are walking this path with you. And it's healthy to be able to give and receive support and to share in a variety of experiences and opinions on pregnancy, birth or parenthood, even if they don't fit with your personal view. Birth-preparation or parenting-preparation groups are great places to meet like-minded couples who are going through very similar experiences. Often friendships made in groups like these can last way into your child's lifetime.

Take a moment now to appreciate your current community, your existing family, friends and people who enrich your life. When you have done this, reflect on what aspect of your community you might want to develop, or what kind of networks you might like to be part of as you parent your children.

Appreciate your community, your family, your friends and the people who enrich your life

List any antenatal classes or groups that you are attending, or plan to, and any new friends you make along the way.

Weeks 13 & 14

By now your babe-to-be is developing a sophisticated nervous system, and a little face with a chin and a broad forehead that can wrinkle up. Their lips can move and they are starting to practise their sucking reflex as well as their swallowing and breathing reflexes, with amniotic fluid. They grow to between 7.5 and 8.5 centimetres in length and from 23 to 43 grams in weight.

And how about you? How are you feeling? What has been happening in your life? Please tell all...

Who have you told about your pregnancy so far? How did they react?

Food

If you are feeling like you could eat for the Olympics now, and from a much wider range of foods than in the previous few months, it could be time to look for a healthy pregnancy diet that appeals to you and offers optimum, balanced nutrition for you and your growing babe-in-utero.

ESSENTIAL NUTRIENTS

Now is the time to eat fresh and nutritious food, avoiding processed foods and stimulants like coffee and alcohol. There are also a few essential nutrients that need to be included in your diet, such as good-quality vegetable oils (rather than highly saturated fats) as they are high in polyunsaturated fatty acids, which are essential to foetal development. Docosahexaenoic acid, or 'DHA', is an omega 3 fatty acid that is found in cold water ocean fish, seeds and nuts, and has been found to play a critical part in foetal growth, especially in the development of the central nervous system. Oily sea-fish like salmon, mackerel or sardines provide a good source of DHA, or you may want to get your omegas from uncooked pressed oils such as olive, pumpkin seed, hemp, sesame, sunflower and starflower or from blends of these that are high in omegas 3, 6 and 9 so that you can optimize your baby's health and your own as you eat.

BLOOD SUGAR LEVELS

It is also especially good to keep blood sugar levels steady in pregnancy by eating smaller amounts of naturally occurring sugars – such as fruit, maple syrup, honey – rather than cane sugar or refined fructose. The main reason for this is because the placenta acts as a filter to ensure that your baby-in-utero receives what they need to function and grow, such as iron and insulin, even if that means that YOU have less of them. Therefore, we often have less insulin in our blood during pregnancy, which can be diagnosed as Gestational Diabetes. This is a temporary condition, which simply means there is not enough insulin needed to use and to mobilize the current higher levels of glucose in our blood. This condition normalizes after birth, but it does mean we are better off eating foods with a low glycaemic index, cutting out pure sugars and getting enough exercise in pregnancy. A low-sugar, yeast-free diet can also help to manage the thrush (yeast infections) that many pregnant women experience.

BE KIND TO YOURSELF

Ultimately, it is good to have a kind relationship with yourself around food, so remember if comforting eating for you looks like a tub of ice cream, maybe you could curb that habit a little to look something more like an exotic fruit salad? There is a big difference between 'comfort' and 'body-kindness' when it comes to what we eat. Maybe you could explore this a little through journaling.

What are you craving right now?

....

....

....

....

....

....

Are you getting plenty of fresh fruit and vegetables?

....

....

....

....

....

....

....

Do you feel that you receive enough vitality and nutrition from the food you eat?

....

....

....

....

....

....

....

....

....

....

If not, then what could you let go of and what could you have more of?

Expand on these questions as much as you like...

Weeks 15 & 16

Your rapidly growing little one is starting to move around in the amniotic fluid of your womb. They can now make faces and begin to grasp their umbilical cord as well as sucking their fingers. That is pretty exciting! They grow to between 10 and 11 centimetres in length and from 70 to 100 grams in weight.

This is also the time that many mothers have a first scan of their baby-in-utero. If this is you, then please share your experience and how you felt. You could attach your scan photo into your journal on the opposite page if you like, to make your memory more vivid.

And do share anything else that has been lovely or significant to you in whatever way during these weeks.

Stress

Lots of stress is one of those things that doesn't compliment women's hormonal functioning at all and is best avoided in pregnancy. Reducing stress now will ultimately be reducing stress later in childbirth and new motherhood, which is the best gift you can give both yourself and your baby. Obviously sometimes stress is unavoidable, but if and when it can be side-stepped, then this is a good time to think about how.

The following pages are for you to consider exploring any ideas for potential changes to your lifestyle that will significantly support your deeper needs for minimizing stress. For example, if you are working in a stressful job it might be worth thinking about whether to speak to your employers about how your stress could be reduced at work or even to organize an earlier maternity break. You could reflect on the causes and origins of any stress you generally have, on a day-to-day basis, thinking about what triggers and pressurizes you.

You may come up with some solid ideas about adjusting your weekly schedule to decrease those tense moments, but it's also good to remember that sometimes it is not the activities themselves that create pressure in our lives, but our approach to them. If you are a 'late' person, you might feel stressed-out just being late for everything. Giving oneself extra time is so helpful! Certain lifestyle practices, such as mindfulness, are also hugely helpful for reducing tension in our lives – I can't recommend meditation enough for women in pregnancy. And another big part of stress-reduction is making time for relaxation and exercise, so this space is for your musings on this subject...

What can you do to relieve any current stress in your life?

Weeks 17 & 18

Your babe now grows to between 13 and 14 centimetres in length and from 140 to 190 grams in weight. They have been practising breathing with amniotic fluid for a little while now and soon begin to rehearse digestion and excretion, also using the amniotic fluid surrounding them, which travels in through the mouth and is passed out through the bladder. Baby's hearing is just becoming fully formed, so this is a lovely time for you and your partner to start talking or singing to them, or playing them music.

These are big developments for your little one, but how about you?

What developments are happening in your life?

How do you feel as you stride into your second trimester?

Worries

Worry is like stress on the inside, and who needs it, right?

The truth is that once we start to focus on doubts and fears they can just grow bigger and bigger, until they take up far too much room in our thoughts and our lives. But even so, it can be really worthwhile to acknowledge them from time to time, just to air them and to release the tension we may have been feeling about them.

Sometimes pregnancy can bring worries to the fore. There are so many themes that might potentially worry us, everything from perceived issues about our growing baby-in-utero, to our birth or feeding choices. These uncertainties might be based on our own beliefs or perhaps they derive from the opinions of others. Either way, they can be equally unsettling. So how do we manage this phase of life without letting fears take over?

It's always worth asking yourself whether or not this is a matter you can actually do something about. If it is, then simply do it and try to let it go. If it isn't something you can act on and your anxiety persists, my feeling is that it could be helpful to explore it here in this journal and/or with a friend who is good at listening with an open mind. And beyond that, just be extremely kind to yourself and find ways to relax when you notice you're worrying. If your worries are overwhelming, you could try working with a therapist to address these issues.

We all worry and it is totally natural, but it does bring more tension into our lives. If we can learn coping strategies to handle this in pregnancy we will probably become more relaxed mothers in the long run. Breathing deeply and counting slowly to 10 can be useful to temporarily settle the mind.

Use these pages to air some of those nagging worries or concerns you may have and think about how to approach them in a way that creates more calm for yourself.

Weeks 19 & 20

Baby's eyelashes, eyebrows, fingernails and toenails are forming now. She or he will grow to around 15.5 to 16.5 centimetres in length and from 240 to 300 grams in weight. A girl baby's uterus and ovaries are in place, complete with all of the eggs she will have as an adult – isn't that amazing? – and her vaginal canal is forming.

FIRST FLUTTERS

If this is your first baby, you will now start to feel their little fluttery movements in your womb from time to time. If you are a mother already, you may have felt them sooner. So this is a fine opportunity to write about this experience.

What is it like?

....
....
....
....
....
....
....
....

How does it make you feel?

....
....
....
....
....
....
....
....
....
....
....

Do you feel closer or more connected to your little one because you can physically feel them now?

....
....
....
....

_____

_____

_____

_____

_____

_____

_____

_____

_____

_____

What else is going on for you, and what has been happening during these weeks?

_____

_____

_____

_____

_____

_____

_____

_____

_____

_____

_____

_____

_____

_____

_____

_____

Take some space to reflect on this time...

Weeks 21 & 22

Your baby-in-utero has developed soft little hairs all over their skin from head to toe, which is now covered in a protective oily, waxy substance called vernix. Although their eyes still can't open yet, they can hear things both within and outside of your womb. Boy babies' testicles start to move down into their scrotum now, and by the end of week 22 your baby will be around 27 centimetres long and will weigh up to 430 grams. This is also a time when your increasing overall bodyweight – baby included – and womb-size can start to stretch muscles and sometimes cause aches and discomfort.

At this stage of pregnancy, your baby can hear things both within and outside of your womb

So what are you noticing?

....

....

....

....

....

....

....

....

....

....

....

....

....

....

....

Any changes that feel new?

....

....

....

....

....

....

....

....

....

....

....

....

....

....

....

How are your energy levels?

How is your general outlook?

Weeks 23 & 24

From here onwards the cortex part of your baby's brain, associated with conscious thought, starts to develop more and more. They can now sense if they are upside down or not. Their muscles and all organs are also continuing to grow and mature rapidly and they grow to around 28.5 to 30 centimetres in length and between 500 to 600 grams in weight.

Taste buds have formed on their tongue, their bone marrow now begins to make blood cells and they have found a rhythm of sleeping and waking regularly and even have REM when dreaming.

And on that note, have you been writing any dreams down? Your dreams can be very vivid at this time (see page 12), so do include the details of these if you remember them.

How are you feeling in yourself?

Can you remember any recent dreams?

Weeks 25 & 26

Your baby's reflexive movements increase and they now start to fill out a bit more, storing body fat and still growing strong. They will range from around 34.5 to 35.5 centimetres in length and 660 to 760 grams in weight.

Although they cannot open their eyes yet, they will soon be able to sense light from behind their closed lids. At this time babies can start to respond to sounds around them and a loud noise might make them move suddenly. This is a special phase when you and your baby can sense and respond to each other.

Have you felt your baby respond to sound?

How are you feeling?

Weeks 27 & 28

You may be feeling that your body is taking on an entirely different shape now as that beautiful and 'definitely pregnant' roundness comes into fullness.

Meanwhile, your baby's head-hair is growing and the 'hand and startle reflex' develops in their movements. Their growth ranges from around 37.5 to 38.5 centimetres in length and 875 grams to 1 kilogram in weight, and all the while they are gaining more weight.

But how are YOU doing? Please tell all...

At this stage, your beautiful and 'definitely pregnant' roundness comes into fullness

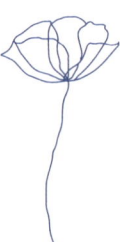

What are your favourite things to wear at the moment? Is there anything that's difficult to wear?

The Second Trimester is Complete

Week 28 marks the end of the second trimester, a significant time!

You are drawing closer to the final few months of gestation and to the birth of your child. This is a moment to acknowledge the last few months, starting with any problems or difficulties and moving on to all that you feel thankful for at this time and some celebration! You are amazing! Keep that in your heart and mind.

What has been challenging for you?

What are you truly grateful for?

What would you like to celebrate?

THE THIRD TRIMESTER

During this final stage of pregnancy, your baby will be going through different developmental processes and refining of their senses, organs and bodily functions in readiness for birth and life beyond the womb. You may already be noticing a range of movements from them, including kicking, stretching, rolls and hiccups. These will be easier to sense when you're resting. This is a fascinating time in many ways, as the little person inside you becomes more baby-like, with their own more conscious experiences that you can share in part but not yet fully. You begin to get to know them from an intuitive and sensory place, but this is still the prologue of your child's epic story that will go on for many, many, many chapters!

It would be lovely if you could make a note here of any observations you've made about your babe's activities so far.

When does your baby tend to be awake – in the day or night?

....

....

....

....

....

....

....

....

....

....

....

When do you notice their movements?

....

....

....

....

....

....

....

....

....

....

....

....

....

....

....

What kind of movements do they prefer to make?

Are there any other interpretations or intuitions you've had?

Preparation

The third trimester is also a time when your pregnant body will really feature centre-stage in your life as you experience growing your child into all their fullness within the home of your womb. Many women really enjoy this time of ripening. And yet still there will be times when the stretching, the swelling or the weight of your body will be uncomfortable. This phase will bring its inconveniences, just like the first trimester. If this is the case, at least you know that it is only a matter of weeks until your body changes again and pregnancy gives way to motherhood. The other thing about these last few months of pregnancy, is that they hold the quality of 'unknowing', i.e. when your baby will arrive, what your baby will be like, how the birth will go, and so on. Some women are at ease with this scenario and others aren't. I think it can be helpful to think of this final phase as a time for gently getting practical things in place first and 'nesting' so that you don't have to rush to do them at the last minute. It is also helpful to do what preparation you can now to make your birth, postpartum and newborn time more relaxing and enjoyable.

Why not write a list here of the practical essentials you want to complete alongside a list of things that might seem like extras but which might be valuable assets in making your birth and new mothering experience a really lovely one, which is just as important.

In the third trimester, you experience growing your child into all their fullness within the home of your womb

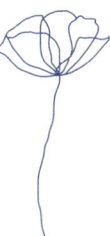

What essential things do I need to organize now?

What other things can I sort out if I have the time and energy after the essentials?

Weeks 29 & 30

By now your baby's eyelashes are complete and their eyes will be starting to open a little. Their central nervous system has become sophisticated enough to maintain their body temperature and to direct regular, rhythmic breathing movements. Their growth ranges from around 38.5 to 39.9 centimetres in length and 1.2 to 1.3 kilograms in weight.

Your uterus is now moving higher up in your body, between your ribs and your belly button. You might experience some itchiness on the skin of your belly as it stretches. Unblended oils like almond, coconut or olive oil massaged gently into your skin can bring helpful relief, as can washing with fragrance-free soap.

Think about your current needs and wishes, then use this space to write down your thoughts.

Also, think about looking ahead a little and putting some treats in place for yourself.
A massage, some help at home, a daily nap, or anything that makes things easier for
you while you carry your baby-in-utero for these last few months will feel like a godsend.
What could you put in place now to help later?

Have you started 'nesting' yet?

Baby Names

This could be the time to start thinking more seriously about baby names. If you know your baby's gender then you may be ahead of the game here, but either way, you could use this space to list names of either gender, or gender-neutral names, that you'd like to try out on your little one when they arrive.

Keep a list here...

Make a note of any family names that you are considering choosing.

Do you and your partner have different lists? Write some of their preferred names here.

Weeks 31 & 32

Your baby matures and develops more reserves of body fat. Their growth ranges from around 41.1 to 42.4 centimetres long and 1.5 to 1.7 kilograms in weight. You might notice that they are kicking more at times as they exercise their muscles. Baby's brain is developing rapidly at this time, too; their eyes can focus now and their hearing is acute.

Meanwhile, your body will be growing bigger and heavier as you accommodate your baby's increasing size. If this begins to affect your sleep at night, try giving yourself plenty of space in bed and experimenting with positions and pillows in different places – under your bump, between your knees, and so on – to support you.

Sleep will also be aided by making sure you have enough exercise in the day and even trying relaxation techniques before bed or a bit of yoga stretching. Just go easy on your amazing pregnancy-body as you keep in shape.

Try relaxation techniques before bed or a bit of yoga stretching

Perhaps you could share here some of your experiences of sleep and comfort or discomfort, and what works for you?

What kind of movements is your baby making?

Is there anything else that feels significant for you at this time in your pregnancy?

Weeks 33 & 34

Your babe is continuing to gain weight and although all of their major organs are fully developed now, their lungs still need to mature a little more. The vernix on their skin thickens to prepare and condition their body in readiness for birth. As they grow to around 45 to 46.2 centimetres in length and 1.9 to 2.1 kilograms in weight, they have less room to move around, which can mean that they're a bit less active. You may take more notice when they do move around, according to your own position or activity or the sounds around you.

With baby taking up more inside space and pressing against your stomach, you may find that you get heartburn or reflux from time to time, especially after a meal. Avoiding acidic or deep-fried foods, fizzy drinks, caffeine, red meat and alcohol can help with this. Remember to keep pampering yourself! And do write about your feelings, your thoughts and everything that's been going on for you during these weeks.

What's been happening during these two weeks?

....
....
....
....
....
....
....
....
....
....
....
....
....
....
....
....
....
....
....
....
....
....
....
....
....
....
....
....
....

How have you been feeling?

Have there been any big changes?

Birth Wishes

This is a great time to start noting down your birth wishes if you haven't already. You could think of it like an invitation for your health-care provider to support you in the way you'd like to be supported during and post birth. Whether you are planning to give birth in a hospital, at a birth centre or at home, think about who you'd like to have with you and what kind of 'vibe' you want in your environment – for example, tea-lights, birth pool, music, massage, attendees whispering, etc. It's also helpful to include your preferences around medical interventions and your wishes for: Plan A, Plan B and possibly a Plan C, too.

There are so many resources out there to help you structure and flesh out your birth wishes, so do a bit of research before starting as it may save time (also check the reference section at the back of this book).

Think of your birth wishes like an invitation for your health-care provider to support you in the way you'd like to be supported

If you can find one in your area, some couples choose to have a Birth Doula or Postnatal Doula present either during or after birth, or both, and the birth outcome statistics on these assisted births are very positive. Whoever you want at your side, just make sure that they are on the same page as you, that they understand your wishes and that they can stay calm and relaxed throughout, however birth unfolds.

It's worth keeping in mind that childbirth can unfold in many different ways and it does help to be flexible and open to change. If your birth partner can assert your wishes during birth, then you are more at ease to be in your flow and just to go with it.

So on that note... what are you planning?

Explore your feelings about various medical interventions.

Do you have a labour playlist?

Weeks 35 & 36

This is getting exciting! Many babies will have manoeuvred themselves into a head-down position by now, but there is still plenty of time for them to shuffle around if they haven't got there yet. They adopt the traditional foetus position, curled up with knees against chest, but can still move and stretch around. If you are going to birth-preparation classes, your antenatal teacher may have some helpful ideas about exercises or postures to encourage baby into a good position for birth.

At this time they grow from around 46.2 to 47.4 centimetres long and between 2.4 to 2.6 kilograms, so you may be feeling more tired with a lot of your energy going towards nourishing your baby and carrying their increasing weight.

Try to find moments to rest in the day during these last few weeks of pregnancy, especially if you are a mum already. Things get pretty busy when baby arrives and it is good to get in your quota of relaxation in before that happens! Think about your needs at the moment and how these could be met.

How are you feeling?

How are you feeling about the birth?

Use these pages to ruminate and reflect on what life is like for you just now.

Weeks 37 & 38

Okay, baby is laying down their body mass, the lovely insulating fat that will help them to stay bonny and well beyond birth. Their growth ranges from around 48.6 to 49.8 centimetres in length and 2.9 to 3.1 kilograms in weight, and just when you think your belly can't grow any bigger... it does!

Your babe is getting ready, how about you? This is when many pregnant women like to socialize less and take some space for themselves. Your focus may become more centred around your home environment as your nesting instinct kicks in and your physical mobility is weighed down. Resting with your feet up is really essential now. Sitting and sipping tea while daydreaming is a wonderful practice for this stage in pregnancy. If you do a lot of cooking, try making meals that are quick to prepare and can sizzle away in the oven so you that you're not on your feet too much, but keep up the gentle strolls outside and yoga or other birth-preparation exercises for movement, if you can. This can also be a time when emotions are more heightened as your hormones get going and birth seems so near and yet so far, so please be compassionate with yourself.

How have you been feeling?

What has been occupying your thoughts? Note down any vivid dreams you have had recently.

Weeks 39 & 40 +

Well, it could happen any time!

Baby keeps growing from around 50.7 to 51.2 centimetres in length and 3.3 to 3.5 kilograms in weight.

How are you feeling Mama? You might find you are tripping over your words a bit, forgetting things and generally being a space-cadet... it's the hormones, not you! And it will last for a while longer as you nurse and raise your baby. Other more instinctual parts of your brain are taking over and getting you ready for birth, and that is perfect. Just don't attempt bookkeeping or scientific analysis of anything right now because they might not work out!

Some women love being pregnant and don't want it to end, ever. Others can't wait to get back to being singular and just to have their baby with them at last without the added weight, strain and complexities of carrying a baby on the inside. And all of these feelings are completely natural.

How are YOU feeling?

Do you feel ready to give birth?

Are your pre-birth needs, like rest and relaxation, being met?

How does your body feel?

Are you excited about meeting your little one?

YOUR
BIRTH

Okay, let's assume that by now you have all the practical
stuff ready? And the rest is a guessing game, a time of
waiting and preparation. Here are a few top tips for birth
that you might want to mull over.

Love vs Stress

The most valuable thing that a woman who is about to give birth
can do, is to create feelings of love and relaxation both in and around
herself as much as possible, and let go of worries or fears as best she
can, to minimize her levels of stress hormones during pre and early
labour. Because relaxation and joy will assist the secretion of oxytocin
as labour approaches. Oxytocin is a core player in the biochemical
team of hormones that carry labour towards full dilation and beyond
birth to breastfeeding (if you choose to) and bonding with your baby.

Oxytocin, the 'love' hormone, which is secreted by the posterior
pituitary gland in the hypothalamus or 'back brain', is stimulated by
empathy, laughter, hugging and breastfeeding as well as physical
touch, orgasm and sensuality. Feeling happy, at ease and 'in love' are
oxytocin-rich states. On the other hand, stress hormones like adrenalin
stall our body's secretion of oxytocin, except in the final stages of
labour when a surge of adrenal-type catecholamines accelerates the
birth process and helps you to push or ease your baby out.

Feeling free to move your body as you choose during birth can really help. Circling the hips is great! Having some music on and slow dancing with your partner can be fabulously oxytocic, especially in early labour. Some women like to be massaged. If you think you'd like this, there are also some excellent acupressure points you could find out about (see reference section), which are believed to support labour and reduce discomfort. Dim light also helps your body to secrete melatonin, which assists the whole birth process, too. It might sound funny, but maybe you could even think of labour as an unusual and intense hot date? This is possible in most settings, including hospitals, if labour progresses normally. Do put it in your birth wishes and make sure the medical staff know that you'd like to be in a calm and intimate birthing environment.

Breath

By listening to someone's breathing, you can tell if they are relaxed or not, right? And when we breathe calm, deep breaths we can regulate our whole physical system, heart-rate and pulse, helping us to release stress and relax. Focused, calm breathing is a great tool in childbirth. Counting through each breath can also be a fantastic way of focusing your mind at moments of intensity. Long exhalations also help to reduce the build-up of lactic acid, which creates the *runner's stich* type cramping around the womb. Practising breathing in for 4 and slowly out for 8 is excellent preparation.

Birth Affirmations

You may find that having a birth 'mantra' or affirming statement can help you to create a positive mindset, bringing focus and relaxation to your birth. Here are a few examples:

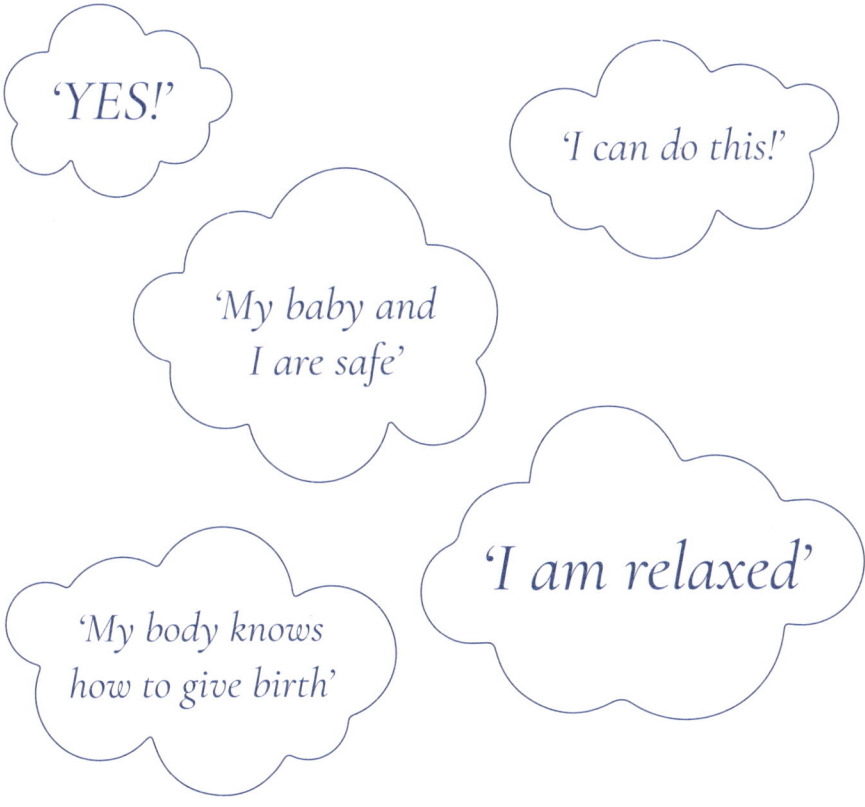

'YES!'

'I can do this!'

'My baby and I are safe'

'I am relaxed'

'My body knows how to give birth'

This may or may not be your cup of tea, but it might still be helpful to use this space to explore your personal thoughts on staying focused in labour or to create some affirmations to support your sense of calm, strength and wellness as you give birth to your baby.

How can you stay calm and focused during labour?

What affirmations could you use?

Sustenance

Dates are now known to be the food of late pregnancy and labour. Apart from the fact that they contain many minerals, amino acids and helpful energy in the form of fruit sugar and protein, it is believed that dates also cause cervical dilation because they contain a compound that mimics oxytocin. The advised quantity is 6 dates per day for the last 6–4 weeks of pregnancy. In fact, dates in combination with coconut water, which has great isotonic properties, is probably the best available team for keeping up energy and hydration levels during labour and if you have these with oatcakes and plain water you have a good GI balance, too. If labour lasts a long time, try and get a few easy, sustaining bites like soups or smoothies in there, too.

What foods will you eat during labour?

Golden Hour

And at the end of it all... your BABY arrives!

So, if everything runs smoothly with the birth, you can make the first hour of their life a gentle, nurturing time for skin-to-skin bonding and generally admiring your divine new family member. If this sounds like your thing, you can add your claim for this 'Golden Hour' into your Birth Wishes, so that whoever attends knows in advance that you'd prefer this to be an un-rushed time, and that mama and papa want to go slow and get to know their newborn. You can check the reference section at the back for more on this theme.

What do you want to happen during your baby's first moments?

This Golden Hour can
be a gentle, nurturing
time for skin-to-skin
bonding with
your new baby

POSTPARTUM AND THE FOURTH TRIMESTER

The physically intense experience of childbirth and the arrival of a new baby into our lives, represents one of the most profound transitions that a woman can make. Mothers are SUPERSTARS! However your birth unfolded, WELL DONE YOU!

The first three months of your baby's life are often referred to as the fourth trimester because they represent an important stage of adjustment for your child, between life in your womb and life outside. It is just as important a time of adjustment for parents (and existing siblings, too) and can include equal measures of sweetness and sleepless chaos.

It is good for a mother to practise 'receiving' from everyone else at this time and not to feel that she needs to play the hostess or look after others. Second-, third- or fourth-time (or more!) mums might struggle with their instincts to continue with their job of care-taker, and it is not easy to stop when you have other children with ongoing needs... but still aim to take a back seat if you can, at least for the first few weeks post-birth, if not longer. In so many traditional cultures all over the world, mothers are fed, massaged and generally cared for after giving birth for a month or more. So do be sure to allow others to look after you. After all, you are the Mothership, you are keeping a small person afloat and you need to be well cared for.

This is also a time when it will be very unlikely that you'll find even a moment to write in this journal! So parts of this chapter are structured in such a way that you can just add your glimpses of this precious time into themed sections. And if some of those journal entries are made when your babe is a year old, it doesn't matter, just use the space as and when you wish to.

Unpacking your Birth

Having just said that a new mum is strapped for time, this bit is really important. See if you can put aside an hour or even half an hour to be alone when your newborn babe is sleeping or being cared for by someone else, so that you can just fully focus on recording and exploring the birth experience you've had. As you write, try to pause to allow any feelings to arise without judging or censoring them. Give yourself permission and time to feel what you feel and allow space for everything that comes up for you. Keep writing until you have communicated whatever needed to be said or written and you feel that for now, you have explored all of the practical and emotional aspects of this memory.

Sometimes there are complications in the birth process or a baby might arrive prematurely. If you've had a difficult time and it feels too challenging to do this alone, I would consider doing an exercise such as this with a loving friend, family member, Doula or counsellor as part of your healing process.

And try to find a way to really celebrate yourself as a mother, be it the birth you had envisioned or not. YOU are truly amazing!

My birth story:

Your Body

General post-birth physical care, except for post-Caesarean surgery, can include gentle belly massage with arnica oil on strained muscles, especially after a warm bath or shower. Foot and leg massage can also be very grounding and nourishing post-birth, and if you are breastfeeding it is good to work on releasing tension in the neck and shoulders.

If you have had an episiotomy or tear it is also helpful to make a tea or use a tincture of calendula and hypericum and add it to your daily bath with a couple of drops of tea-tree or lavender oil to help the wound heal. Finding comfortable ways of sitting that avoid placing pressure on your vagina and perineum is important, too. A doughnut-shaped cushion is often recommended to protect you as you heal, but I think lying down a lot is a great option, too. For post-Caesarean births you need to wait for a few weeks before you can have a long soak in the tub, but do check with your health-care provider about when you can bathe again.

In the Indian Ayurvedic tradition, women practise wrapping a long piece of cloth around their 'empty' bellies after giving birth, and traditional Mexican practices also involve wrapping a mother's post-birth body using scarves in key areas, such as her belly, as it draws the pelvic area back in. You might want to try something similar yourself, but this doesn't work if you have had a Caesarean birth as you need to avoid pressure in this area until your body has healed. Gentle daily exercise is an all-round winner for mothers post-birth.

So how is your body feeling now? You can go into detail on this one, from head to toe!

How are your general energy levels?

What physical nurturing are you enjoying most, such as food, baths, or massages?

What do you need for your own personal healing? What would help you most?

New Mama Food

It is really important to eat and drink well in the weeks following birth, especially if you are breastfeeding. Nourishing protein-rich foods and filtered or spring water are key to maintaining good health while the body adjusts to its new rhythms.

TOP TIPS

Foods rich in iron such as meats, dark green vegetables, pumpkin seeds, apricots and so on are excellent after birthing and if you have experienced any bleeding at birth you could also use a natural iron supplement. Taking in an extra 500 calories daily is also recommended if you are breastfeeding.

Eating easily digestible foods that make you feel nourished is important, so that your digestive system isn't working too hard to do its job, as the rest of the body is still healing from birth and may also be producing milk.

Listen to the kinds of food that your body takes in effortlessly and to those that it doesn't and follow your nose. For me, fresh chicken soup with vegetables is one of the easiest meals for my body to assimilate and it leaves me feeling well-fed. And liquid-rich soups are good for hydration also as they include salt and water at the same time.

Try eating a few olives or something a little salty before drinking water to help the body to hydrate and absorb the water you drink. Coconut water is also excellent for any breastfeeding mums to stay hydrated, and peppermint, nettle and fennel tea all support milk production. If you need any further help with breastfeeding, please see the links to organizations in the back of this book.

What foods are you enjoying at the moment?

What are you craving?

What do you need to eat/drink more of?

Maybe use this space to keep a note of any new recipes you have tried:

Baby Blues

The quality of your post-birth time will depend a lot on the sleeping patterns, emotional states and physical needs of your babe and yourself. If you have a good support network around you it makes everything much easier! But for most of us, it can be said that parenting babies and young children is one of the most rewarding and steepest learning curves we ever face in life.

'Baby blues' is a name given to the time when a mother's first breast-fluid, called colostrum, is replaced by her milk, which 'comes in' two or three days after she has given birth. And, as with all physical changes that are guided by the hormones, things can get pretty emotional. And that's okay! In fact, the whole first year after childbirth can be an emotional time for mothers. We have a lot to manage, looking after ourselves, our babies and often others, too. And doing all of this when we are probably sleep-deprived, it is no wonder we feel a lot.

This kind of emotionality is normal and is not an indication of postnatal depression, but if you are concerned that you might be depressed, please read the section on PND at the back of the book. And do make sure you get some physical and emotional nurturing at this time. Please use this space to write about any emotional, physical or practical challenges you may be facing...

What emotional challenges are you facing?

What physical challenges are you facing?

What practical challenges are you facing?

What do you need help with?

Beautiful Baby!

So, it's 'hello beautiful' to someone tiny and special!
Welcome to the world little one!

What are you like?

How is it for you getting to know your amazing parents?

And how are those amazing parents of yours doing?

Well, I imagine your life may have been turned upside down with your
newborn here now. There will be those endless, blissful moments
of sinking into a loving gaze with them or watching them sleep, or
just holding them and feeling the love. And then there will be times
when they cry or have wind or can't sleep and we may get woken up
and anxiously be trying to work out what they want or need. Often
mothers instinctively know that they are either hungry, in pain or want
a cuddle. If a cuddle doesn't work, we try milk and if that doesn't work
we know that they are most likely in discomfort of some sort (including
tiredness) and we can try to address this.

The reality is that this newborn phase of life will include all the joys
and all the challenges together, in one little bundle. And here is the
space for you to record it all (when you get a moment). Let's start
here with all of your observations and feelings about your baby. Write
everything about them, how they look, their smell and the sounds they
make, etc. You can include your experience of bonding with them, too.
Treat it as an early days diary to record every moment of your first
weeks as a mother.

DATE:

DATE:

DATE:

DATE:

DATE:

DATE:

DATE:

DATE:

DATE:

DATE:

DATE:

DATE:

DATE:

Baby's Changes

A baby changes so radically from day 1 throughout their first year of life, that it can seem fast and slow at the same time. Slow, because everything becomes focused on their rhythms and needs, yet fast because they do make dramatic leaps and bounds and suddenly they no longer fit their Babygro's or they start crawling without notice!

Keep adding to your journal entries as the weeks and months go by, observing your baby's developments and changes, their first smiles, when they learn to roll over, what they're like in the bath and other memorable milestones, and try to include some of these special events here so they won't ever be forgotten.

Include some special events and changes here so they won't ever be forgotten

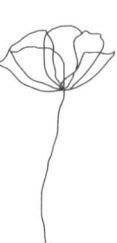

DATE:

DATE:

DATE:

DATE:

DATE:

DATE:

DATE:

Golden Moments

Life with a baby is full of these! Think about those magical times when your baby charms your parents, in-laws, relatives or friends for the first time. It is often so heart-warming and also comical at times to see elders and babies together. Or introducing your little one to their siblings, cousins and other children and seeing their responses and the games this initiates. Babies are so little but they can really have an impact on their surroundings!

You can include lovely events, cosy days or sun-drenched afternoons, funny episodes and poignant moments. Try and capture those moments that you want to treasure and remember from these early days.

DATE:

DATE:

DATE:

DATE:

DATE:

DATE:

DATE:

DATE:

You & Your Partner

By acknowledging yourselves as parents, you can mark the positive beginning of this journey together with your new child and it is important to really celebrate each other. It might be as simple as saying 'YES! We did this!' and 'We are doing this!' and recommitting yourselves to each other with a kiss.

However you choose to honour your parenting bond together, remember to keep your relationship alive as and when you can. It might not be until baby is three months old that you have your first date, and your baby might be the little gooseberry who just happens to be with you on that occasion, but do make romantic moments to land together and share your hearts. Like plants, relationships need nurturing and warmth. Baby will be needing these things too, mainly from mum, but if everyone can be patient and giving, then there will be plenty to go around.

You could use this space together to write what you love and admire in each other, and to share your gratitude for each other as people and as parents...

It is important that you and your partner really celebrate each other

Love

Parenting is like a banquet of soul food that can both challenge and inspire us! It can be a rocky road at times and at others, it is the greatest thing that could ever happen to anyone on Earth. When we realize that the entire journey revolves around love, and occasionally we have to dig around for a good while to find that love, it simplifies everything.

Why not use this last space in your journal to write about what you are loving in your life right now.

I wish you all the very best on your way!

POSTNATAL DEPRESSION

The 'Baby Blues' in early motherhood is quite different to postnatal depression. There are many differences, but the plainest is that if you're really not enjoying your baby or new motherhood, it could be that you have PND. If so, do reach out to others even though that might feel really difficult. There are amazing organizations I've listed in the reference section who would be a great starting point. And please don't blame yourself, because postnatal depression is a state caused by our body-chemistry and if anything, it involves managing one of the hardest challenges that any mother could face.

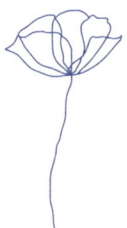

If you have PND, then having people come in to help you in the home environment can really help you to feel supported, and can give you a chance to rest. Exercise is also good for helping with depression as it builds up the body's natural levels of endorphins, it oxygenates the body and it generally refreshes your whole being. Obviously the extent of your exercise will depend on how you are healing physically from birth, but when your body is ready, it is a must. And keep reminding yourself that day by day you are, and you will be, getting better.

Sending you hugs!

You are an amazing mother!

RESOURCES

Pregnancy reading for parents

The Positive Birth Book, Milli Hill (Pinter & Martin, 2017)
Ina May's Guide to Childbirth, Ina May Gaskin (Bantam Dell, 2003)
Mindful Pregnancy & Birth, Riga Forbes (Leaping Hare Press, 2017)
Men, Love & Birth, Mark Harris (Pinter & Martin, 2015)

Doula organizations

DOULA UK
www.doula.org.uk

EUROPEAN DOULA NETWORK: DN
European-doula-network.org

DONA INTERNATIONAL
www.dona.org

AUSTRALIAN DOULAS
www.australiandoulas.com.au

Birth links

spinningbabies.com
activebirthcentre.com

ACUPRESSURE
Debra Betts – acupressure in childbirth, acupuncture.rhizome.net.nz
To download her free booklet, visit
acupuncture.rhizome.net.nz/download-booklet/

Birth wishes templates

The Positive Birth Book by Milli Hill
www.lamaze.org
www.nct.org.uk

GENTLE CAESAREAN BIRTH PLANS
www.motherlove.com/blog

SEEDING A BABY'S MICROBIOME AT BIRTH
The Microbiome Effect, Toni Harman & Alex Wakeford (Pinter & Martin, 2016)
Documentary film 'Microbirth' at **www.microbirth.com**

Golden hour

choicesinchildbirth.org
www.bellybelly.com.au
magicalhour.com

Breastfeeding

Ina May's Guide to Breastfeeding, Ina May Gaskin
(Pinter & Martin, 2009)
The Food of Love, Kate Evans (Myriad Editions, 2008)
The Womanly Art of Breastfeeding, La Leche League International
(Pinter & Martin, 2010)

Breastfeeding support organizations

UK
www.tongue-tie.org.uk
www.abm.me.uk
www.laleche.org.uk
www.breastfeedingnetwork.org.uk
www.nct.org.uk
www.nationalbreastfeedinghelpline.org.uk

USA
www.lllusa.org
www.pebblesofhope.org
www.breastfeedingusa.org
www.naba-breastfeeding.org

INTERNATIONAL
www.llli.org
www.breastfeeding.asn.au
www.lalecheleague.org.nz
www.babyfriendly.org.nz
www.waba.org.my

For multiple births

www.raisingmultiples.org
www.tamba.org.uk/Parent-Support

Postnatal depression support organizations

UK
www.mothersformothers.co.uk
www.pandasfoundation.org.uk
www.nct.org.uk
www.pni.org.uk
www.bestbeginnings.org.uk

USA
www.postpartum.net
www.crisistextline.org
www.maternalmentalhealthnow.org

INTERNATIONAL
www.panda.org.au
www.pnd.org.nz
www.mentalhealth.org
www.mentalhealth.org.nz

For Fathers-to-be

www.fatherstobe.org

Meal planner for friends and relatives to pamper you post-birth

www.takethemameal.com

INDEX

About the author

Riga Forbes is a mother, doula, complementary therapist, artist, and for over a decade has taught Birth Vision courses which support women to prepare for birth mindfully, using meditation, movement, and creativity. Riga has practised Buddhist Vipassana meditation and worked in the healing arts for over 20 years, offering workshops in both Australia and the UK. She has two children, and is the author of *Mindful Pregnancy & Birth* (Leaping Hare Press, 2017).

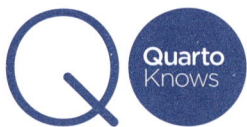

Brimming with creative inspiration, how-to projects and useful information to enrich your everyday life, Quarto Knows is a favourite destination for those pursuing their interests and passions. Visit our site and dig deeper with our books into your area of interest: Quarto Creates, Quarto Cooks, Quarto Homes, Quarto Lives, Quarto Drives, Quarto Explores, Quarto Gifts, or Quarto Kids.

First published in 2021 by Frances Lincoln
an imprint of The Quarto Group.
The Old Brewery, 6 Blundell Street,
London N7 9BH, United Kingdom
www.QuartoKnows.com

A catalogue record for this book is available from the British Library.

ISBN 978-0-7112-6225-6

10 9 8 7 6 5 4 3 2 1

Design by Sarah Pyke

Printed in China

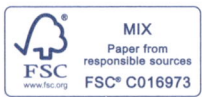